Get Off Your Ass & Mow The Grass!

G. Scott Graham

True Azimuth Coaching

Copyright © 2016 G. Scott Graham All rights reserved

No part of this book may be reproduced, or stored in a retrieval system, or transmitted in any form or by any means, electronic, mechanical, photocopying, recording, or otherwise, without express written permission of the publisher.

ISBN-13: 9798413932971

Printed in the United States of America

Contents

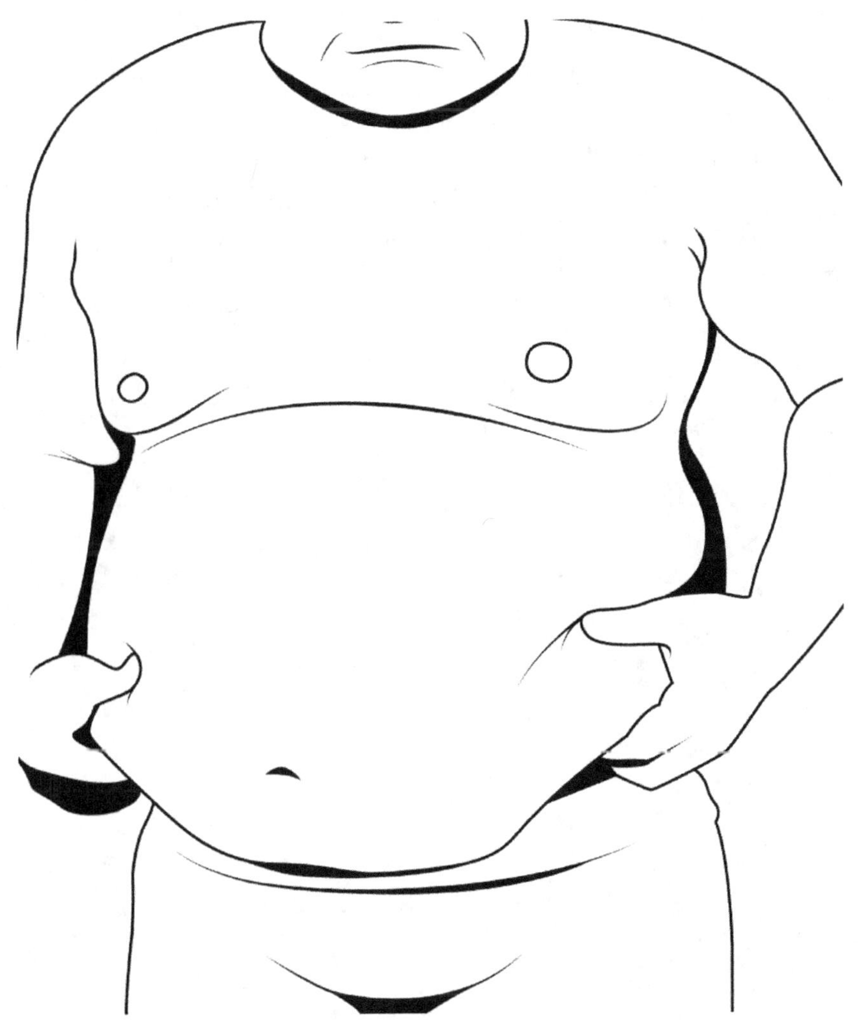

Introduction

"Modern society has done us in. We are surrounded by conveniences. We have machines that wash our clothes, wash our dishes, and wash our cars. We have remote controls for everything from our televisions to our lights. We don't have to move anymore."

G Scott GRAHAM

Seventy-five years ago, we had to walk to the store and lug the groceries home. Seventy-five years before that we had to make most of what we ate. Seventy-five years before that, if we didn't grow it or hunt it, we didn't eat.

Now we can order food right from our smart phones and companies will deliver them right to our front door. We just pop it in a machine, hit a few buttons, and we have our food.

Most people don't grow or hunt for even a tenth of what they eat. We have become consumers. And by 'consumers' I don't mean 'eaters'. I mean consumers in the truest marketing sense. We consume what companies peddle and market to us. And what do they market to us? Crap. Because that is what we buy and that is what we eat: sugar-coated crap.

So, we sit around, hypnotized by advertising, eating what is marketed to us, not what we are hunting and growing, waiting for it to be delivered to our doorsteps and getting fat.

Now you might think this book is about the marketers out there and how evil they are and how you are a complete and utter victim.

It's not.

Because you have a choice.

You have a choice to be fat, get diabetes, heart disease, and die an early death.

It's not genetic.

It's laziness.

It's a habit (and not a good one).

And you don't need to get gastric bypass surgery.

And you don't need to join a gym.

You just need to get off your ass and start moving around.

You are probably familiar with the phrase 'thought-provoking.' The Merriam-Webster dictionary defines thought-provoking as "causing people to think seriously about something" (and I hope this book is thought-provoking).

In that same sense I want to introduce two new phrases into our language:

- Fitness-provoking and
- Fat-provoking

Fitness-provoking is defined as "causing people to get serious about their health and fitness" while fat-provoking is defined as "causing people to ignore their health and fitness."

The solution is simple. It's not rocket science: you need to practice more fitness-provoking behaviors and fewer fat-provoking behaviors.

The Riding Lawnmower

There is no invention of modern society that is more fat-provoking than the riding lawnmower. As a personal trainer and health coach, there is nothing I find more disturbing than seeing a fat person mowing their postage stamp-sized suburban lawn astride a riding mower.

I suppose it could only be worse to see a fat person sitting on their deck, drinking a weight loss shake while they watch someone else sitting on a riding lawnmower mowing their lawn.

Really?

Get off your ass and mow the grass!

G. Scott Graham
December 2016

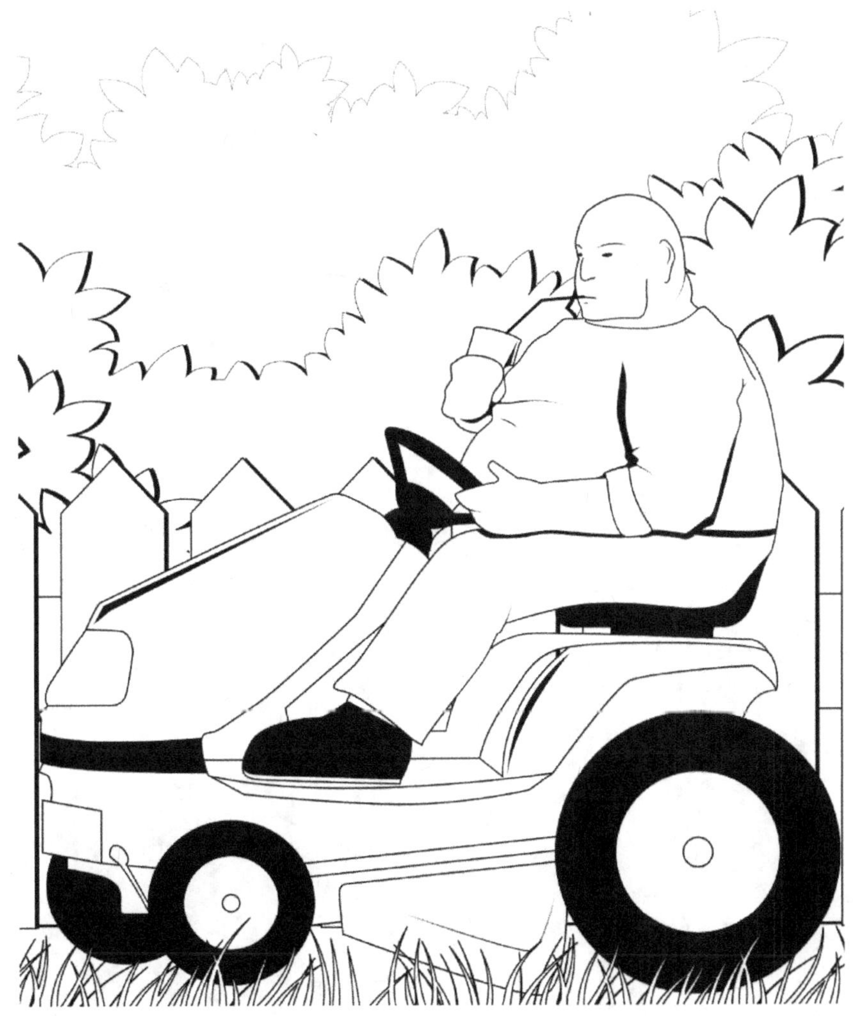

What this book is about

"People are very open-minded about new things - as long as they're exactly like the old ones. "

Charles KETTERING

This book is about one thing and one thing only: **convincing you to sell your riding lawnmower, buy a push mower and invest the difference in a personal trainer or health coach.**

That's it. Not much more.

But, as Charles Kettering astutely points out, people struggle with new ideas. It is hard to be open to new frameworks - especially when they are as radical as the one that I propose in this book.

And make no bones about it, the change I am suggesting is radical.

I know that you have invested a large chunk of change in a riding lawnmower. I know that mowing your lawn is a public exercise and those neighbors used to seeing your fat ass astride a riding lawnmower will wonder what is going on. I know that pushing a lawnmower is not easy (that's why it works, by the way).

These are strong reasons to continue with the same old same old.

These are strong reasons to stay fat.

So, knowing all of this, I realized I had to write a book.

And through it all, I will do my best to convince you to change this one aspect of your life so you can reap the rewards of increased fitness and health.

I will share my own story - an experiment, actually - of how I trained and completed a half-marathon simply by mowing the grass.

And along the way I will share some tips and strategies about fitness, running, mowing, hiring a personal trainer or health coach, and more.

If I am effective in convincing you to switch to the push mower lifestyle, you may even offer to mow your fat neighbor's grass (for a fee) and then invest that money in personal training and health coaching.

And if I am *really* effective in convincing you about this lifestyle, you may even go out and get a reel mower.

Hardcore converts may be inspired to go out and get a scythe…

I have experimented with all these mowing tools over the past years, driven primarily by the rural setting I call home, which is hours from a gym. There are practicalities around time and effort that emerge when you live in the middle-of-nowhere, and you can gain from the wisdom I have gleaned from these practicalities.

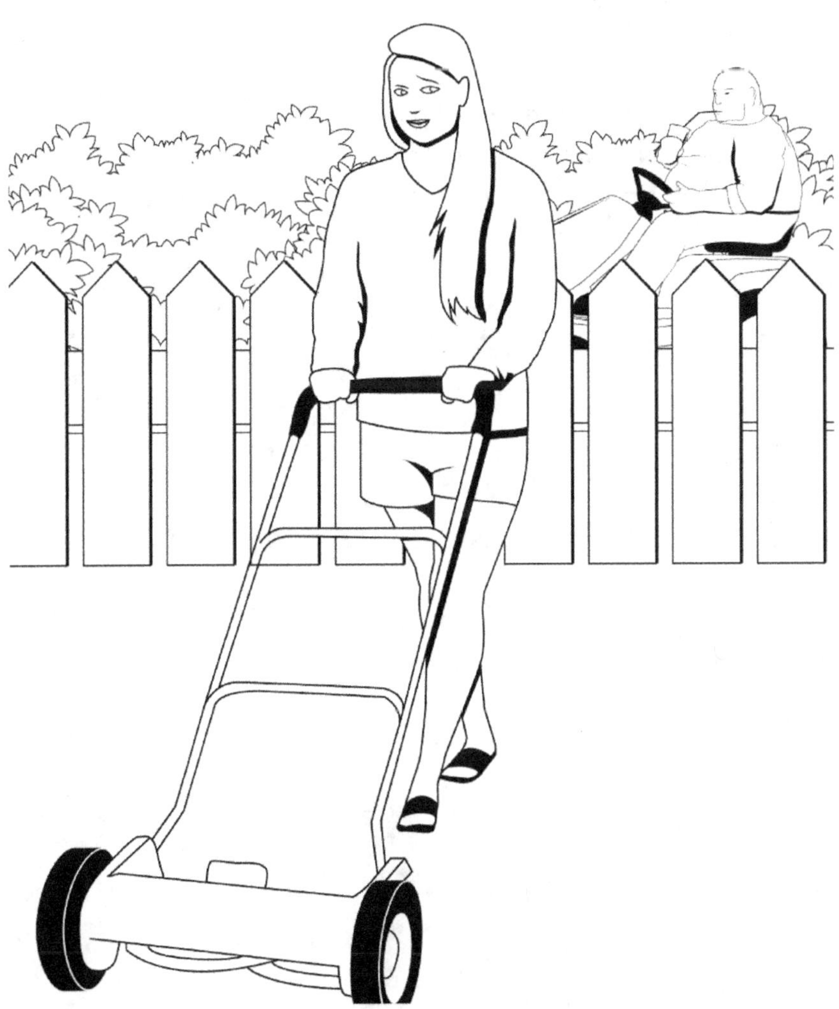

Why do we even need a riding lawnmower?

"An escalator can never break, it can only become stairs. You should never see an 'Escalator temporarily out of order' sign, just 'Escalator temporarily stairs. Sorry for the convenience.'"

Mitch HEDBERG

don't get it. I just don't get it.

Well, I could understand if you had acres to mow (although I do mow my TWO acres by reel mower and scythe with the assistance of a few sheep and alpacas).

But less than two acres?

Why would you get a riding lawnmower if you had less than two acres?

Does it save that much time?

The truth is that a riding lawnmower does not save that much more time than using a push mower.

Sure, if you are a professional and mow lawns for 8 to 10 hours a day in the summer, you probably own one of those zero-turn stand-behind or sit-on mowers that promise 15 miles per hour. But no one - except maybe those folks maintaining golf courses - runs at that speed.

Most non-professional people run their lawnmowers at 4 to 5 miles per hour max. After all, they don't want to run over their fellow family members, pets, flowers, lawn ornaments, small rocks, and a multitude of other obstacles they haven't seen since winter began.

I have news for you: 4 miles per hour is walking.

Now you may be thinking, "But my riding lawnmower has a much wider cutting area than my push mower." That is true. You may gain a few inches with each passing swipe on the lawn, but will that amount to hours saved by riding instead of walking?

The Race

I am naturally curious. So, my spouse, Brian, was not surprised at my suggestion of a race as part of the research for this book. He would ride proudly astride a riding lawnmower and I would humbly but confidently use a push mower (not self-propelled).

The first task was to find the proper parcel of land worthy of the competition. This was no small task. After all, we do live in Vermont. There's not much flat space and there are lots of rocks that pop out of the ground like toadstools each spring. After much debate, we finally agreed that we would not be able to compete at the same time: in order to be fair, we would mow the same parcel of land. Each trial would be timed and the time compared to determine the winner.

Having decided on the course, we now turned our eyes to the tools of combat. We no longer had a riding mower so we looked to borrow one. Luckily, we live in a world full of fat people who spend time on riding mowers so we didn't have to look far.

We engaged a mutual friend to be referee and judge. He methodically took three samples from the emerald blades of grass so as to correctly assess the height and dispense with any accusations of bias, inconsistency or foul play that might be raised by the losing party.

We also agreed on the following rules:

1. No running
2. Starting the mower would not be counted in the timing
3. We could move forward or backward over the grass to deliver the decisive slices to our quarry
4. The clock would stop when the mower was put away and the mowee (as to distinguish from the mower) walked across the finish line (we wanted to minimize the risk for any injuries at the very end of the competition, driven by some mad dash to victory)
5. Time would be added to a participant's total for sloppiness and missed sections at the discretion of the judge

The three of us surveyed the agreed-upon course, which was straightforward and included an open area, an area around some plantings and a line of shrubs that needed to be cut as close as possible.

One might have been tempted to label the course as favoring a push mower, as the person astride the riding lawnmower needed to make some fairly tight turns as well as maneuver their beast of a machine in some smaller spaces. The course, however, also included an open area on a slight hill which could arguably put the push mower-wielding contestant at a disadvantage.

We drew straws and Brian would go first. He mounted his steed and started it up.

He chose to circumambulate the entire course twice before beginning his sweeps back and forth from end to end. Because of the tight quarters, he was forced to go slowly and work methodically so as not to miss a blade and have a penalty added to his final time. Like a Buddhist practicing walking meditation, his concentration was focused and his actions were purposeful. Unlike the Buddhist, however, enlightenment and mindfulness were far from his mind. His concentration remained unbroken throughout, his eyes on the prize: Brian was focused on winning. Period.

After a few minutes his strategy was clear: he had eliminated all the complex maneuvers that would be required on the course and had an open space where he could "open her up" and speed to victory.

I watched the clock worriedly as he zipped back and forth from end to end, aware that Brian was making a heck of a time to beat when it was my turn. He seemed like an obsessively neat locust, speedily and oh-so-exactly consuming his helpless grassy prey.

As he completed his last run, Brian now turned his focus to parking the mower in the garage and then crossing the finish line. He put the mower in neutral and turned it off, dismounting the mower while it was still rolling forward like a stuntman exiting a moving vehicle. He approached the identified finish line, the porch.

It took him a total of 33 (nail-biting) minutes and 15 (agonizing) seconds to complete the course.

And now the verdict: the judge began his survey. To practice his art to the best of his ability, he insisted he complete it in privacy, so we both waited on the front porch while he walked the perimeter of the course, clipboard and tape measure in hand.

He returned a few moments later, a serious look on his face, to announce that he had added two minutes to Brian's time.

We had agreed beforehand that we would not demand an explanation concerning any allocated penalties in an effort to avoid debate, discord, and to preserve our friendship. The final official time for Brian's run was 35 minutes and 15 seconds. That was the time to beat.

We adjourned and now all we had to do was wait. And wait. And wait. (Would the wait ever be over?)

I never fully appreciated the idiomatic expression, "it's like watching the grass grow" until now.

We figured it would be a week, so planned to meet up and measure the grass seven days from Brian's run. But we had no rain. None, nada, nichts. So, the grass had hardly grown in seven days' time.

We waited two more days. Then one more. Then another.

I used each passing calendar day to strategize, then analyze, then assess, then problem-solve and strategize again. After all, there was a lot **riding** on my performance. Fat people the world over would feel vindicated in sitting on their asses all summer long if riding indeed proved to be a significant time saver.

I needed to win. Or at least come in close to Brian's time.

And I had faith that I would do so. I had been practicing fitness mowing for some time and knew from my direct experience that the time compared to using a riding mower was not significant. But this was a timed experiment, one that would be featured in the book if I performed well and that would spell the demise of the book if I performed poorly.

Finally, on the morning of day thirteen, our friend, our judge, our referee announced (hallelujah) that the grass had grown to be equal in length as it was on the day of Brian's run. It was my destiny to take on the course tonight.

At four o'clock we reconvened.

I started my mower and awaited the signal from the judge. I hoped I had chosen my weapon carefully, deciding against a self-propelled mower on the assumption that I would save precious time not having to stop and change gears.

"Go" reverberated in my head as I launched into a not-running-but-almost-kind-of-walk that was my offering in the face of the challenge. I heard the objection from Brian that I was running and I countered that I was merely **walking quickly**. My strategy was different than Brian's. My goal was to maximize the lawnmower moving backward. I also made a trim line along the garden so I could start there and work my way forward, so that the last cut I made was closest to the garage where I would eventually need to store the mower (see! That strategizing while the grass was growing came through!) I made short order out of the tight back section that took Brian so long to maneuver around and went directly on to the area requiring wider cuts back and forth alongside each other. This was the section in which Brian performed outstandingly and I was determined to minimize things like turn time which I noted had added time to his total. So, I simply pulled the mower behind me for each row. I was determined to win. Similarly, the hedges posed no problem for me as I simply eased my way down among them, back and forth with the mower.

I finished that section and then moved on to the final patch which, like the area I attacked first, required some small (but mighty) ninja moves.

I finished and quickly headed toward the garage.

I had kicked ass. I knew it. I didn't even need to look at the time.

I turned the lawnmower off while I was pushing it toward the garage, gave it one big heave ho when I was about 15 feet away and turned toward the finish line. I stepped up on the porch and turned to note that the push mower was sitting nicely in the garage as I heard my time: 30 minutes and 30 seconds.

"Ha!" I thought. Wait until people read this in the book!

Then I looked up and felt my stomach drop.

You could see it from the porch. Easily. You didn't even need to walk over to know I had missed a wide swath of grass. I may as well have missed an area the size of a football pitch.

In my oh-so-clever-rush to pull the mower behind me and save time, I had lost track of where I was and at one point simply missed that grass. Had I taken the time at the very end to quickly survey the competition area I would have seen the patch crying out to be mowed. I would have been able to cut it and most likely matched or still even beat Brian's time. But in my arrogance, I didn't even look. How could I be such a fool!

Our judge / friend grabbed his clipboard and surveyed my mess while Brian and I waited on the porch for the verdict.

He returned a few moments later, again a severe look on his face, to announce that he had added six minutes to my total time.

I had lost.

Or had I?

Brian's time was 35 minutes and 15 seconds. My time was 36 minutes and 30 seconds.

Although I technically lost – a state of being that I think I am genetically pre-disposed to bear harshly – I had shown that there is not a huge time difference between pushing your way to fitness or sitting your way to fatness via your lawn.

Time was not, and is not, an issue.

Now I could explore the other parts of the equation: calories and money.

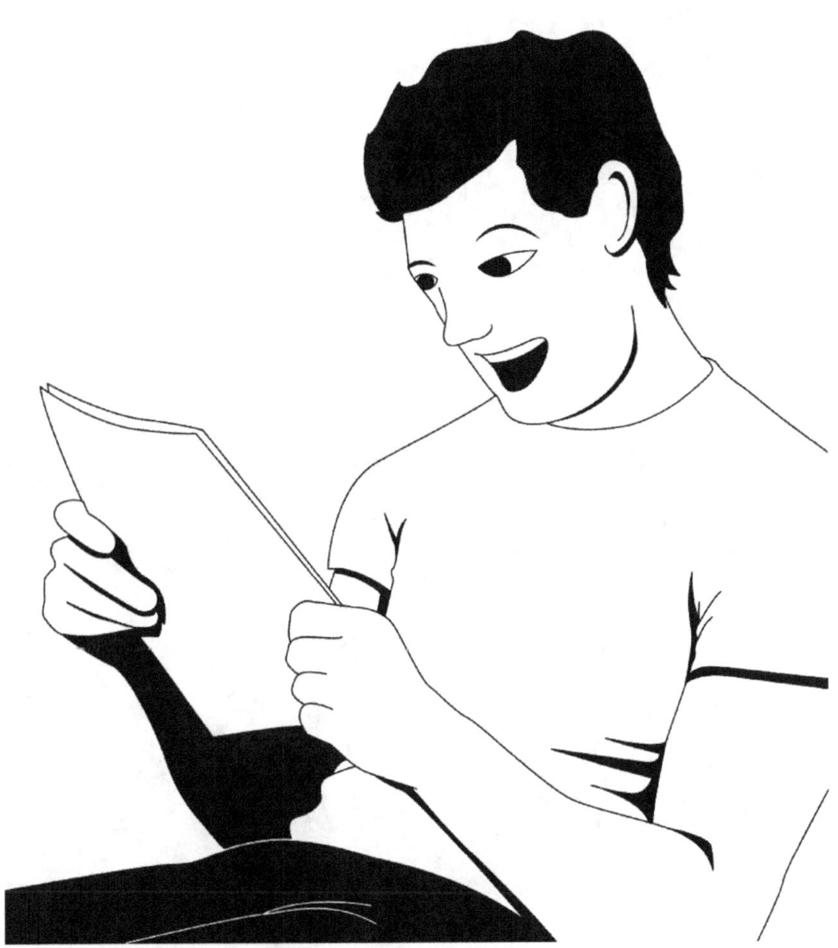

Look at the facts. Do the math

"Everyone is entitled to his own opinion, but not his own facts."

DANIEL PATRICK MOYNIHAN

The Calories

Now that we have dispensed with **time** as the factor in why anyone would mow their lawn with a riding lawnmower instead of a push mower, we can take a closer look at what your choice to sit on your ass instead of exercising is costing you in terms of calories.

How many calories do you burn whilst mowing the lawn, riding that mower for one hour? Approximately 86 calories. If you decided to do that same lawn walking behind a power mower you would burn off 202 calories in that same hour. That's an increase of 135% in calories burned in the same time period! Opt for a non-power-driven mower (you know, one that you actually push?) and you will bump your caloric burn to 288 for that hour or a 235% increase!

There is no other exercise switch-up that I know of that can yield those results!

Imagine the impact of spending roughly the same amount of time mowing the grass that you are **already** doing but burning almost two and a half times more calories!

Want to really give yourself a workout? Go get a reel mower (you know, one of those that has no engine at all!) and you will expend 458 calories or an increase of 433%. That's almost four and a half times more calories!

Here's a Summary Chart:

	Calories	Percent increase over riding
Riding mower	86	
Self-propelled	202	135%
Push mower	288	235%
Reel mower	458	433%

The Money

Well, I hope these numbers have convinced you of the value of getting off your ass and pushing your way to better health. But just in case they haven't, let's spend some time on cash. Cold hard cash.

Cash speaks loud and clear to a lot of people. So, if I failed in convincing you to get off your ass and push a mower about your lawn for health reasons, maybe you'll consider doing it for the money.

I don't want to turn this book into a math class. So, you will have to trust me that I have done the math correctly and accept these facts as presented. Let's take a look at the financials for these four mowing choices:

- A reel mower will set you back anywhere from $70 to $150.
- A gasoline-powered push mower will set you back anywhere from $150 to $300.
- Make that gasoline-powered self-propelled and you can expect to pay $250 to $500.
- Decide to sit on your ass and purchase a riding mower and you will pay between $1,000 and $3000.

But the story doesn't end there. Most people today buy things on credit. So, let's say you have $100 in your pocket and you decide to get a mower. You can pay for the lowest priced reel mower outright and still have $30 in your pocket.

If you decide to get a gasoline-powered push mower you will have to finance $50 for the base model and $200 for the top of the line. If you manage to pay $25 per month you will pay off the lowest priced model in about 2 months and will have spent a total of $151.15, assuming 18% interest. Finance the top-tiered push mower and you will pay it off in 9 months and you will have spent a total of $314.65, assuming 18% interest and the same $25 per month payment.

Upgrade to self-propelled and you will have to finance $150 for the base model and $400 for the top of the line. Using the same parameter for financing as we did for the gasoline-powered push mower (18% and $25 per month), you will pay off the lowest priced model in about 6 months and will have spent a total of $258.36 and for the top model expect to pay it off in 19 months and you will have spent a total of $560.82

Now let's run those same numbers for the riding mower. This is where it gets interesting. You will have to finance $900 for the base model and $2900 for the top of the line. Assuming 18% and $25 per month as before, you will pay off the lowest priced model in 52 months and will have spent a total of $1,404. However, at $25 per month, you would **never** be able to pay off your debt for the highest priced model - you would need to pay more than $43.50 per month to manage it. So, at a $44 per month payment, you would pay off the top-tiered riding lawnmower in 300 months and will have spent a total of $13,331.78.

Quite a difference. It's the power of the time value of money working against you.

But what if you let the time value of money work for you? Let's say that instead of buying that top-tier riding lawnmower you invested $70 in the reel mower, put the $30 in an interest-bearing account and then put the $44 you would have paid for the privilege of sitting on your ass into that same interest-bearing account for the same 300 months you would have sent it to the creditor.

Guess how much you would have at the end of that time?

At only 6% interest, you would have $29,990.14 in your bank account.

That's worth noting again: instead of spending $13,331.78 to sit on your ass, you could earn $29,990.14 for the privilege of burning off 433% more calories each hour you cut the grass. That's a difference of $43,321.92!

What would your skinny-self do with that money?

Here's a summary chart:

	Reel Mower	Push Mower	Self-Propelled	Riding
Lowest	$70	$150	$250	$1,000
Payment	$0	$25	$25	$25
Months to Pay	0	2	6	
Total Paid	$70	$151.15	$258.36	$1,404
Percent	**100%**	**216%**	**369%**	**20,006%**
Highest	$150	$300	$500	$3,000
Payment	$25	$25	$25	$44
Months to Pay	2	9	19	300
Total Paid	$151.15	$314.65	$560.82	$13,331.78
Percent	**216%**	**450%**	**801%**	**19,045%**

**Percent refers to ratio of total price of each mower to total price of the base reel mower. To put it in words, the top-tier riding mower costs 19,045% more than the base reel mower.

Note: If you have never thought about the time value of money and these numbers shock you, I suggest you spend seven hours listening to John Cummuta's Speech from Nightingale-Conant, titled, "Transforming Debt Into Wealth: A Proven System for REAL Financial Independence."

John does a great job explaining the time value of money, the lie we have been sold by the credit machine, and how to stop playing that game.

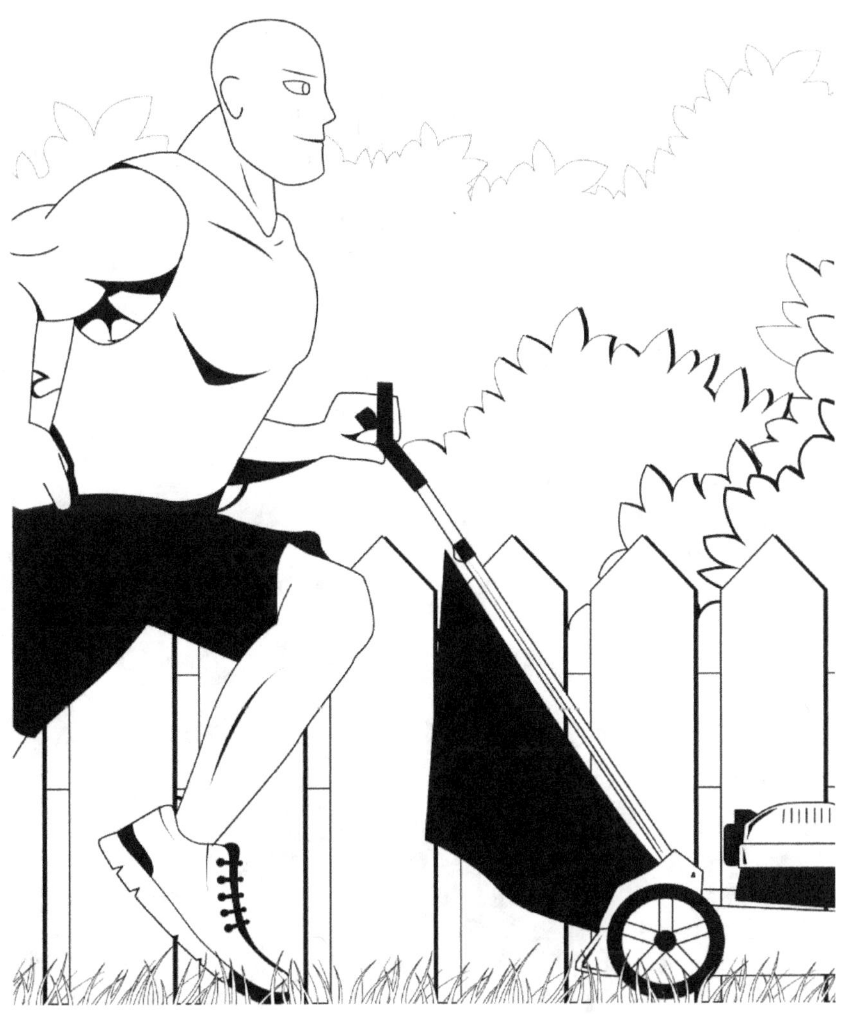

A few thoughts on running & mowing

"Out on the lawns, there is fitness and self-discovery and the persons we were destined to be."

ADAPTED FROM GEORGE SHEEHAN

As a personal trainer and health coach the third biggest mistake I see clients make is that they make the decision to run for exercise and then just start running - the rationale being that they have run before and know how to do it. (You can read about the top five biggest mistakes I see clients make in the Appendix). Well, it is OK to just run - and run fast and hard - if you are running out of a burning building or running away from a bear (though someone once told me back in my days as an Outward Bound instructor that I need not worry about outrunning the bear; I simply had to make sure I outran the slowest person in the group).

But if you are running regularly for exercise, your poor running form and habits will wreak havoc on your bones and muscles. The truth is that most people run incorrectly and then seek out a mechanical intervention (shoes, orthotics etc.) to correct their bad form and bad habits. This is like simply picking up golf clubs, heading straight to the driving range, and then striving to solve the resulting swing and stance problems by purchasing better golf clubs...

If you wouldn't do it with golfing or other sports, why do it with running?

Recommended running strategies

I recommend clients who are starting to run to check out the Galloway Method as well as ChiRunning. These are two complimentary approaches to running:

- The Galloway Method focuses on pace.
- ChiRunning focuses on form.

The Galloway Method

The Galloway method mixes running with walking. You read right. You walk in the Galloway method. But to be sure this is not some scheme where you run until you are exhausted and then walk the rest of the way. You run, then walk, then run again using very specific timeframes.

You decide for yourself what these timeframes are (called intervals) and run / walk accordingly, and you carry an interval timer (which you can get for about twenty bucks) during your 'run' to prompt you to start walking and then start running again. The total time for a complete cycle of one running interval followed by one walking interval is usually between 1 and 2 minutes. And you do this cycle over and over and over again throughout the entire race. You can usually spot the Galloway runners at a 5K, 10K, half-marathon, or marathon because they are the ones that keep raising their right hand (as they move over to the far right and walk) followed by raising their left hand (as the start running again and merge with the other participants.)

Now I have to tell you, when I first heard of the Galloway Method, I gave it zero thought. In fact, I thought it was just bullshit so I completely ignored the concept. But one November at Disney World I found myself squarely confronted with the power of the Galloway Method.

I was doing RunDisney's Wine and Dine Half-Marathon, a night race through three of the parks ending at Epcot on one of the last weekends of the Epcot Food and Wine Festival. Maybe it was because it was dark (the race started at 11:00pm) and there was little else to pay attention to, maybe it was because Disney at night is surreal or maybe it was because I was wasted from running a 5K with Brian 16 hours earlier that same day. Either way, I realized that I kept running past the same couple who were walking. It was apparent because every time I ran past them while they were walking, they said "Hi."

I noticed a pattern eventually. I was trudging on and they would walk then sprint then walk then sprint. I just ran steadily forward. Then something changed. Somewhere around the fourth hydration stop – mile 9 I think - I stopped seeing them. I wondered if they were OK. Maybe something had happened and they had to drop out I worried. After all, I had come to really feel connected to these 'walkers', having hop-frogged them about 40 times. I thought to myself, "They should have prepared so they could run the whole race." An hour later I finally saw them - after I crossed the finish line and was eating a banana. Actually, they saw me and came trotting over. "Great race, eh?"

I asked about their time and just about fainted when they told me. "And you walked?" I quizzed them. "Walk – run – walk," they replied. "Galloway is incredible."

So, in the face of my comparatively pathetic performance, I decided I would give it a try. For my next half-marathon, I trained and prepared in typical fashion except for one thing: I bought an interval timer and set it for 45 / 15, meaning I would run for 45 seconds and then walk for 15 seconds for the entire race. I have to re-emphasize that this is the only change I made. Everything else was the same. I even ate the same food for dinner the day before and wore the same outfit to the race that I donned in the previous half-marathon. I was leaving nothing to chance in my experiment.

The results: I knocked 30 minutes off my time. THIRTY! THIRTY!

I couldn't believe it.

Then another realization hit me. I had done a half-marathon (13.1 miles), knocked 30 minutes off my time - a new personal best - AND I ran for three quarters of the time and walked the rest. "Oh my god," I thought, "I got my personal best and only had to run 9.8 miles!"

That's not really true. Because in the Galloway method, when you run after you have given your legs a 15 second break by walking, you cover greater distances than you would have if you had been continuously running. I probably ran 10.8 miles. Still, that means that I walked 2.3 miles.

I was converted and now when I run a race it is always with an interval timer at my side.

Resources for the Galloway method can be found in the Appendix.

ChiRunning

This experiment got me thinking. If my pacing was wrong - and I mean **way** wrong when changing such a simple thing could knock 30 minutes off my time - what else could I be doing wrong? So, I started reading, skimming, and generally perusing the endless stick of running books on Amazon with an eye for form. I found lots of books that were filled with all kinds of tips for how to keep your feet landing in the right way as well as drills, training regimens, and the lot.

And then, one day, I found the book "ChiRunning." Danny Dreyer (another marathoner like Jim Galloway) promised a "revolutionary method," and the book's description was peppered with phrases like, "run faster and farther with less effort" and "injury free running."

I, of course, thought it was total bullshit.

Then I remembered that I had thought the same of the Galloway method until I was trounced by 'walkers' and knocked 30 minutes off my time when I adopted his method. So, I told my critical voice to shut up and ordered the book.

Now I have to tell you that ChiRunning is not easy to learn and master, especially when you have just been running down the road for your entire life and never thinking about form.

But it is amazing.

I didn't get it from the book. So, I ordered a video. Just as useless.

So, I signed up for a class. That was the ticket.

You see, I needed more than a philosophy and instruction. I needed more than demonstration. I had an entrenched running form that was so whacky (just like everyone else I see who runs races) that I needed feedback and correction. I needed someone to say, "No. Lean forward like this." I needed someone to place their hand on my shoulder while I was leaning against a building and tell me, "This is the form you want to have."

ChiRunning has transformed my running. Not because running is easier.
It is. Not because it is more fun (because it is easier). It is. ChiRunning
has transformed my running by giving me something to focus on while I
am going down the road. Running is no longer some mindless, mp3-
filled activity. I can focus on improving my lean and core one day and
on better use of my arms the next (and that's just the start).
ChiRunning has elevated my running into an art form.

ChiMowing?

In addition to ChiRunning, there is ChiWalking. In ChiWalking you focus
on alignment and using your core just like you do in ChiRunning.

Now I am not going to add a lot here because maybe at some future
time we will see the book 'ChiMowing' from Danny Dreyer (or maybe he
will just edit or advise a rewrite for this section of this book). Who
knows, maybe he will even hold ChiMowing instructional courses out on
some golf course! (I can just picture 20 people with mowers going at
it!). Until then you will have to be satisfied with ChiWalking as a
reference, plus my tips below.

I have been practicing ChiMowing (which is basically ChiWalking
modified to hold on to a lawnmower) and can attest to the following
learnings which will help you out:

- Adding a push mower to the mix will either help your alignment
  (because you have something to lean toward and hold on to) or
  totally derail your alignment (because you are pushing against
  something that has resistance). As silly as this sounds - adding a
  mower to the mix - I had a fear of falling forward into the
  mower and the blade mechanism, and getting chopped up like
  some C-list actor in a bad horror movie. Let me assure you, that
  just won't happen. If you fall forward, you will just push the
  lawnmower out of your way!

- The steady pace of a power-driven mower helps you focus on form. I found it helpful to start off at a slower speed to ensure I got the form down before progressing to faster speeds.
- You will propel a reel mower faster than you ever thought you could and will be a lot less tired if you practice the skills of ChiWalking. I was actually surprised how easy it was to propel the mower forward by not pushing it but by aligning my frame so my body weight did the work.
- The mower itself seems to provide a nice benefit by giving you something to lean toward. I found that ChiMowing actually improved my posture when practicing ChiRunning!

Resources for both ChiRunning and ChiWalking can be found in the Appendix.

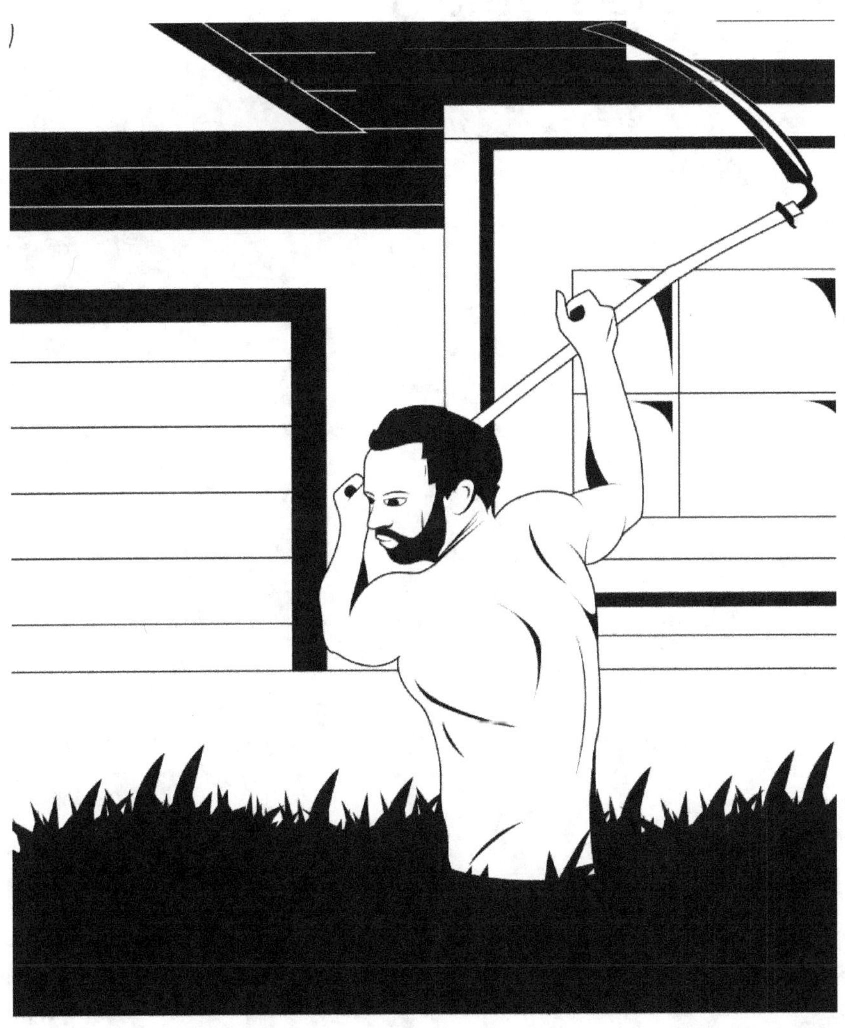

The super-tool to push your fitness level: the scythe

"The tallest blade of grass is the first to be cut by the scythe."

RUSSIAN PROVERB

While writing this book I did a lot of direct research mowing the grass. I had no idea that something as readily available as one's own lawn could create such a high level of fitness if you just embraced it. As part of my own journey to embrace the lawn, I ended up owning two gasoline powered mowers - one that is self-propelled and the other 'Scott-propelled'. Plus, I purchased two reel mowers. After all, how could I expound the differences these tools bring to fitness mowing without using them myself?

Then, one day, I discovered the holy grail of fitness mowing: the scythe. Before telling you about this miraculous fitness tool, let me first educate you about pronunciation so when you talk about it, you sound hip and cool (and that's important). The first half of this one-syllable word seems to be consistently pronounced as in "sigh". Depending on which part of the English-speaking world you come from, however, the second half is either pronounce hard like the word, "the" or soft like the word "thanks".

Now that we have dispensed with the English class, let's move on to the tool itself. First, a scythe is not a sickle. Although they are both used to do similar tasks on the farm, the sickle is a one-handed tool and the scythe is not. You used two hands with the scythe, and you stand up straight when using it (compared to bending over when using a sickle.) Finally, you use your core muscles when scything instead of your upper body / arms when "sickling".

Note: the Grim Reaper carries a scythe (to reap the dead).

You outfit your snath (that's the wooden part of the scythe) with different types of blades (length, material, and thickness) allowing you to tackle everything from light grass to brushy woody plant, and do your scything everywhere from confined spaces (as in the garden or along hedgerows) to ditches to large areas of grass.

I will tell you that scythes are at best perplexing. But, if you embrace this tool, you will soon find yourself, in the words of Pal Joey, "bewitched, bothered and bewildered." I have found the experience fascinating because, as with ChiRunning, I have form to focus on and a technique to perfect. And the feedback you get from the scythe as to whether you have correct form or not is instant and blunt.

Now you may be wondering whether a scythe is effective or not. To answer that question, let me direct you to two YouTube videos – competitions in fact – where you can see how effective and efficient a scythe is:

- Scythe vs Brushcutter 1 - South West Annual Scythe Festival - June 2010, https://youtu.be/gsflHiBB6xE
- BCS mower versus scythe 2012, https://youtu.be/1I4RNenmfFI

There are only two books that you can buy about scythes and scything that I know of. Information on these can be found in the Appendix.

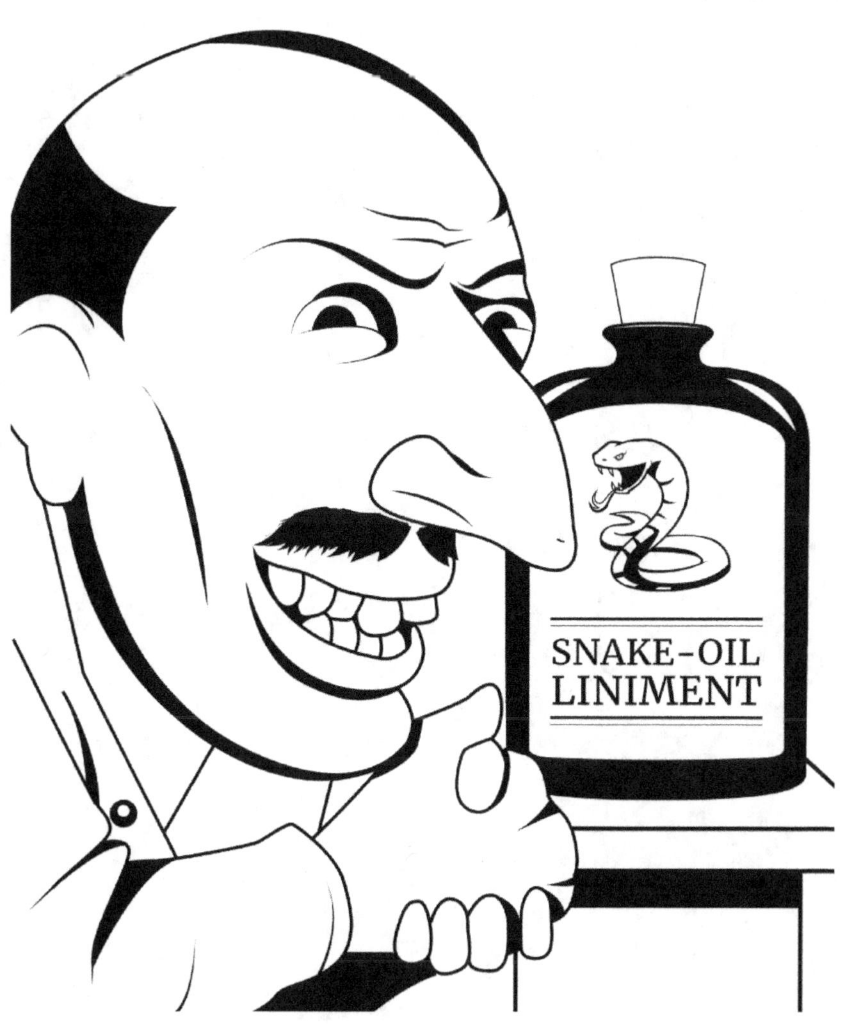
SNAKE-OIL
LINIMENT

Hiring a personal trainer or health coach

"Every swindle is driven by a desire for easy money; it's the one thing the swindler and the swindled have in common."

MITCHELL ZUCKOFF

We now come to the second part of my proposal. You have successfully gotten off your ass, ditched your riding lawnmower, and are actively engaged in fitness mowing. Now, what to do with the money you have saved?

Yep. Get yourself a personal trainer or health coach

Key differences between a personal trainer and a health coach

Personal trainers have been around since there have been gyms to work out in. Initially, personal trainers were the jocks who already worked out at a gym and it was a no-brainer for them to work at their regular hang-out. Over time, personal training became more and more professionalized. Then, in the 1990s, life coaching emerged on the counseling scene. Soon there were many flavors of coach: from ADHD coaches to time management coaches to gay love coaches. You name it, there was a coach for it. Health coaching, wellness coaching, and fitness coaching also emerged as coaching variations and these still persist to this day.

So, what's the difference? To answer that question, I went to the American Council of Exercise. The American Council of Exercise, or ACE, offers both personal trainer and health coach certifications. As part of developing these credentials, ACE has identified Scopes of Practice for each (to a lesser extent for health coaches), as well as minimal requirements for each credential. Scope of Practice defines acceptable behavior for a professional coach.

Personal trainer minimal-certification requirements and Scope of Practice

In order to sit for the Personal Trainer Certification Exam through ACE, an individual must:

- "Be at least 18 years old
- Have completed high school (or the equivalent)

- Hold a current CPR/AED certification with a live skills check."

ACE defines the personal trainer Scope of Practice as follows:

- "Developing and implementing exercise programs that are safe, effective and appropriate for individuals who are apparently healthy or have medical clearance to exercise
- Conducting health history interviews and stratifying risk for cardiovascular disease with clients in order to determine the need for referral and identify contraindications for exercise
- Administering appropriate fitness assessments based on the client's health history, current fitness, lifestyle factors and goals utilizing research-proven and published protocols
- Assisting clients in setting and achieving realistic fitness goals
- Teaching correct exercise methods and progressions through demonstration, explanation and proper cueing and spotting techniques
- Empowering individuals to begin and adhere to their exercise programs using guidance, support, motivation, lapse-prevention strategies and effective feedback
- Designing structured exercise programs for one-on-one and small-group personal training
- Educating clients about fitness- and health-related topics to help them in developing healthful behaviors that facilitate exercise program success
- Protecting client confidentiality according to the Health Insurance Portability and Accountability Act (HIPPA) and related regional and national laws
- Always acting with professionalism, respect, and integrity
- Recognizing what is within the scope of practice and always referring client to other healthcare professionals when appropriate
- Being prepared for emergency situations and responding appropriately when then occur,"

Health coach minimal-certification requirements and Scope of Practice

In order for sit for the Health Coach Certification Exam through ACE, an individual must:

- "Be at least 18 years old and hold a current CPR/AED certification with a live skills check.
- SUBMIT PROOF of one of the following before registering for your exam:
    - Current NCCA-accredited certification or license in fitness, nutrition, healthcare, wellness, human resources or a related field.
    - An associate's degree or higher from an accredited college or university in fitness, exercise science, nutrition, healthcare, wellness, human resources or a related field.
- At least two years of comparable work experience in any of the industries specified above."

Unfortunately, where ACE has done an exemplary job in delineating the Scope of Practice for personal trainers, they have done a pathetic job in doing the same for health coaches. The emphasis from ACE, based on their own instructional materials, seems to be to ensure that health coaches avoid certain areas of nutrition (like meal plans, medications, supplements, and diagnosis) as well as generally not doing anything out of their Scope of Practice which ACE, as I have said, has done an abysmal job of defining.

In my opinion, the work of a health coach consists essentially of the activities of a personal trainer, avoiding infringing on the Scope of Practice guidelines for registered dieticians, plus at a minimum:

- Assessment of motivational and behavioral problems as related to fitness, health, and wellness.
    - Health coaches do not provide diagnoses

- Intervention: use client-centered counseling techniques, such as motivational interviewing, to increase client motivation for change and decrease their ambivalence toward health changes.
- Education and prevention: provide general wellness education.
- Referral: when appropriate, refer the client for additional services.
- Documentation: maintain client documents outlining assessment, goals, and progress for each session.
- Professional and ethical standards: adhere to all ethical standards and applicable state and federal laws, including HIPPA.

How a personal trainer or health coach can help you

A personal trainer focuses primarily on exercise and will help you develop a specific, custom exercise program based on your body (they will assess you) and your goals. They will help you with correct technique, and most importantly will provide you with an increased sense of accountability and motivation.

Using the ACE health coach certification as a framework, the health coach not only can provide these services (after all they need to be a certified personal trainer prior to taking the health coach exam, at least through ACE) but they will also focus on your whole being, including your lifestyle, not just exercise. They will help you set SMART goals (Specific, Measurable, Accountable, Realistic and Time-focused) and by applying counseling techniques, like motivational interviewing, can help you to problem-solve and shift problematic thinking patterns that keep you stuck.

Choosing a personal trainer or health coach

Today, anyone can call themselves a personal trainer or a health coach.

Anyone. In as little as one weekend. Just Google 'personal trainer certification' and 'health coach certification' and see for yourself that people can become 'certified' in the space of a weekend in-person seminar or even in a few hours of home study.

Coaching and to some extent personal training, have become modern day snake oils. Be careful in the choice you make. Caveat emptor.

Note: My dog has two coaching certifications. Yes, you read that right. In an effort to see just how much of a scam the certification industry is, I put it to the test and was able to get my dog certified as (1) a holistic life coach and (2) a relationship coach.

So, what is a person supposed to do?

My best advice is to simply let insurance companies do the work for you. This simply means asking a prospective personal trainer or health coach to show you a copy of their malpractice insurance. Think about it, insurance companies are in the business to make money so they aren't going to provide a million dollars of professional malpractice insurance to someone who has passed the same rigorous credentialing qualifications as my dog.

If you are looking for additional information to help you come to your decision, the criteria outlined in my book, 'Ten things you need to know about coaching before you get a coach', is just as applicable to personal trainers. You can find a link to this, as well as a companion website for the book, in the Resources section in the Appendix.

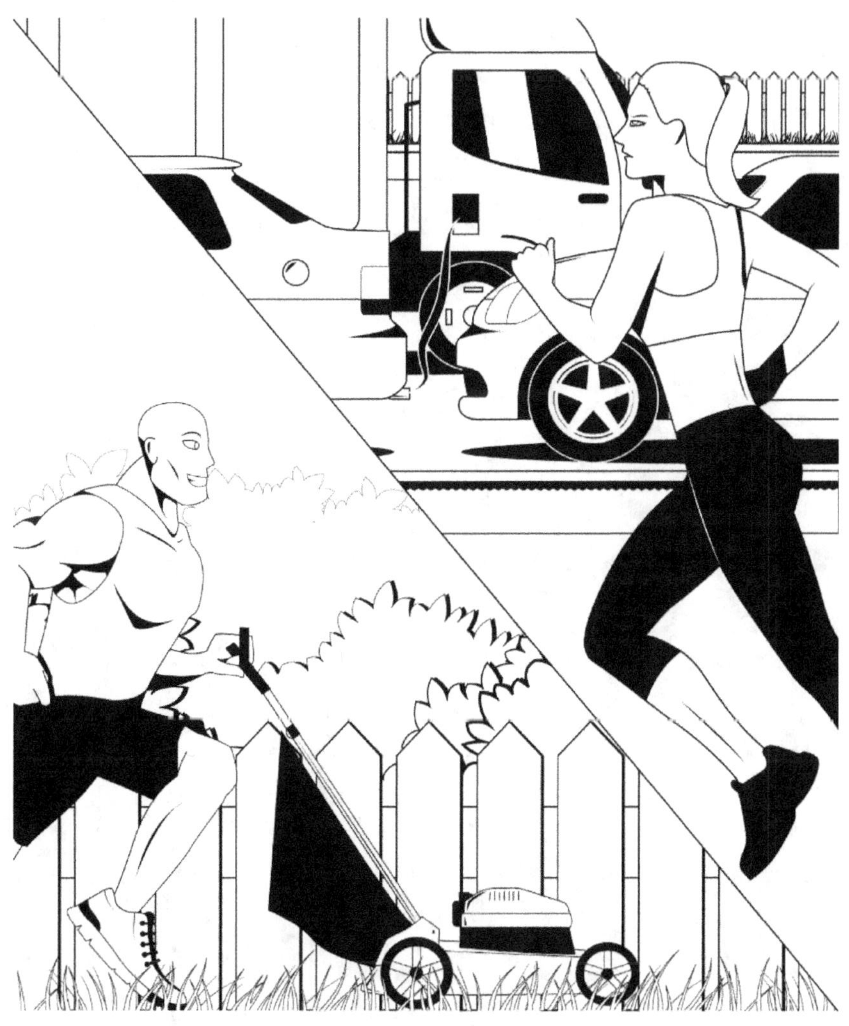

Training for a half-marathon: a story

"Nothing will work unless you do."

MAYA ANGELOU

am the type of person who puts their money where their mouth is.

Sure, a person could lose weight and be healthier from choosing to dismount their riding lawnmower and practice fitness mowing. But could they really develop a high level of fitness from mowing the lawn?

I knew that if I was going to convince people to get rid of their riding lawnmowers and push their way to better health in the summer months that I had to answer this question. Unfortunately, I seemed to be the first one to ask this question. So, I had to come up with the answer myself.

Having trained for and completed a number of half-marathons, I thought, "Could I train exclusively by mowing the lawn for a half marathon?"

As I pondered that question one misty May morning, I felt my stomach churn. The thought of a half-marathon without being prepared for it was troublesome at best and embarrassing at worst. An image of me collapsing at mile 9 and ending up in the Emergency Medical tent flew through my head quickly followed by a mental movie of me telling my friends, family and clients - oh yes, my clients - about my failed attempt and experiment. Not to mention the impact on this book. Mowing the lawn had to produce tangible fitness results. A fitness mowing regimen had to work. I believed it would work. But there was room for doubt.

I finished my coffee and opened up the Facebook app on my phone. I made the bold announcement on my business's Facebook page, then immediately followed it up with a Tweet. Now I had done it. As far as my personality goes, once I put my mind to something there is only a small chance of turning back. Add a public announcement to the mix and there is no - zero, zip - chance of me backing out.

Luckily, I live on a farm. And there are acres of grass to mow. Acres.

Acres on a slight hill.

So, I knew the training course could work.

But it would be once a week or every 10 days.

I silently prayed for a summer with lots of rain.

Mother Nature delivered and, in a few weeks, I found myself mowing a lot.

In the spirit of full self-disclosure, I must report that I did go on various day hikes that summer as I always do. To spend a summer in New England and not stand on the top of at least 10 four thousand footers is just not acceptable. Maybe it was the hikes I took with my father when I was young, or the years spent as an Outward Bound Instructor., but hiking in the woods is a big part of my life.

What I did not do for the three months preceding the marathon was run.

I must, however, again in the spirit of full self-disclosure, report that I did do some sprints while pushing a reel mower. This was actually hard work and one day - due primarily to poor self-care and no stretching (though I should have known better...) - I found myself lying on the ground with blinding leg cramps while my Jack Russell licked my face - pretending to revive me as if I was mortally injured, when really what she was doing was seizing an opportunity to lick my face.

I also employed ankle weights while mowing to add an element of strength training to my mowing.

On average it would take me 5 hours to mow the lawn. Eventually I broke this into multiple days so it actually felt more like running - at least it was distributed throughout the weekly like my runs were.

Finally race day arrived. I had signed up for the Disneyland half-marathon (you must have already guessed that I like RunDisney).

We flew in (from east coast to west) two days before the event in the hopes of minimizing jetlag.

I was nervous. I had no appetite the day before - usually such things are my excuse to consume lots of carbs, despite knowing that carb-loading is just a now-popular myth, fueled by Italian restaurants and pizza parlors. I woke up in the early hours of race day feeling nauseous. Had I prepared enough? Was this folly?

Only a few hours left until the verdict was in and I would be pronounced guilty or not guilty. I could not be presumed innocent. If anything, this could be considered pre-meditated stupidity on my part.

The race went flawlessly until mile twelve. And then I hit a wall.

The last 1.1 mile was excruciating. But I persevered and blasted past the finish line.

Later that day I took the opportunity to debrief the race and ponder what happened. This wasn't the first time that I hit a wall near race end. It could have been the training routine I had concocted with the help of 2 acres of grass. More likely it was the result of the fact that I hadn't eaten as much as I typically would have because I felt nauseous and anxious, so I ran out of fuel at mile twelve.

I had not broken my personal best. But I had finished, absolved of most, if not all, stupidity. And I had demonstrated indeed that fitness mowing is definitely a viable activity, not just for general health, but for serious athletes.

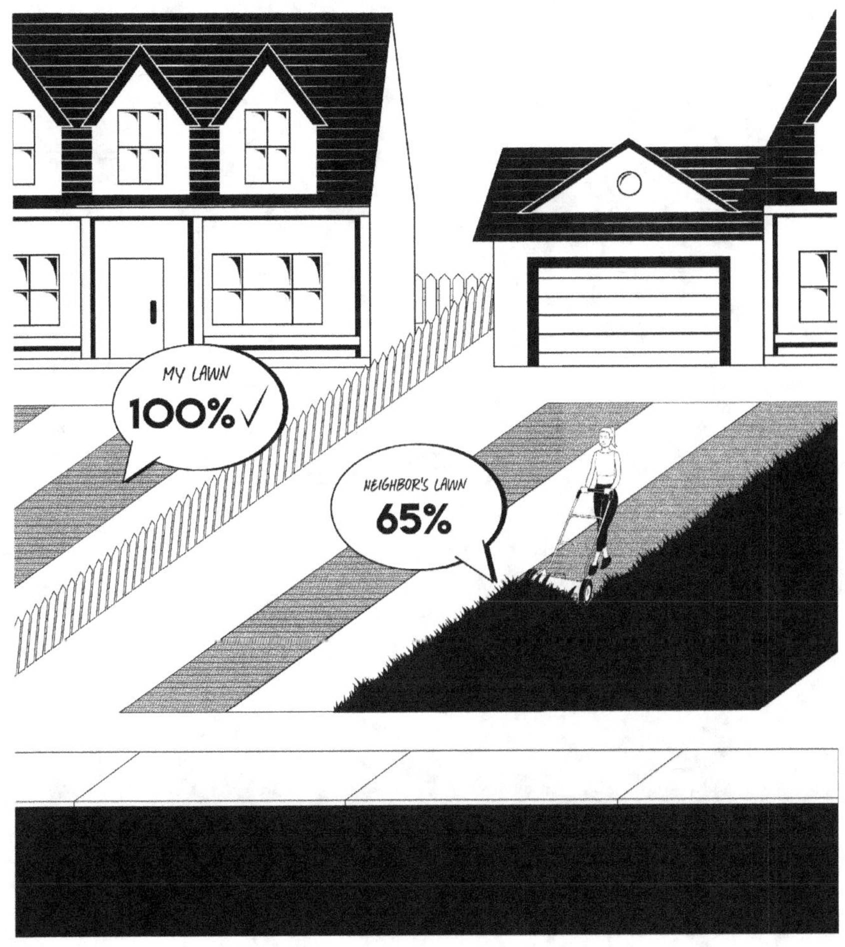

MY LAWN
100% ✓
NEIGHBOR'S LAWN
65%

Final thoughts: consider mowing your neighbor's grass

"A bad neighbor is as great a calamity as a good one is a great advantage."

HESIOD

O K, so maybe I have convinced you to get off your ass and mow your grass but now, as I close this book, I want to suggest that you that you get off your ass and mow your *neighbor's* grass.

"You have got to be kidding," you say.

No. I am absolutely not kidding.

Really, why *shouldn't* you mow your neighbor's grass?

Mowing your own grass is going to get you one day of exercise every seven to ten days.

Well, I have news for you: that is not enough.

If that is not enough, then you have to ask yourself, what else can I do?

First, if you have invested in a personal trainer or health coach, she or he will help you find and clarify that answer.

While you are waiting to get a personal trainer or health coach, I have four options for you:

1.   Buy a bigger piece of property so you have more grass to mow
2.   Walk
3.   Jog / run or
4.   Mow your neighbor's grass

Firstly, let's cross off option one. That might happen next year but if you are wheeling and dealing properties and then moving, you won't be mowing any grass.

Now let's run the numbers and compare running or walking to mowing:

	Time Spent	Calories Burned	Money Made
Walking	1 hour	180	0

Jogging / Running	1 hour	388	0
Push Mowing	1 hour	288	$50

And finally, all you have to do is decide whether you could use some extra cash and what you could do with that extra cash.

Let's do the money like we did in chapter four. Assuming you mow 3 lawns in addition to your own you will average a $125 per week income from May through October. This takes into account some periods where you will mow every 6 days in the rainy spring and other periods where you might go 10 days between mowing.

You are increasing your caloric output to a total of 1152 calories each week.

You toss that $125 in the bank each week and leave it there through the start of October. So, you have 5 months and 20 weeks roughly. At 6% interest, at the end of your summer fitness mowing program, you would have $3,050.50

What would your skinny-self spend that money on?

Appendix

"Appendix usually means, "small outgrowth from large intestine," but in this case it means, "additional information accompanying main text." Or are those really the same things? Think carefully before you insult this book."

PSEUDONYMOUS BOSCH

Stretching

Stretching is important even when you are "just mowing the grass". Stretching is good period, so to include it in your grass-mowing regime would be good for your health.

Pushing and pulling a lawnmower puts a strain on your shoulders and your core, so it's not about just stretching your leg muscles.

The following stretches will help prevent injuries.

For detailed instruction on stretching, I recommend the book, Full-Body Flexibility by Jay Blahnik.

Top 5 mowing stretches

Quad Stretch

- Stand with your feet about hip width apart
- Put your left hand on your lawnmower (or other stable fixture – chair, tree, wall) for balance
- Bend your left leg so that your heel moves toward your backside and grasp your foot in your right hand
- Lean slightly forward
  - You should feel a stretch in your left quad
- Hold this stretch for 30 seconds
- Repeat with the other leg

Calf Stretch

- Find a wall
- Stand arm-length away, facing toward the wall
- Stand with your legs staggered so that your right leg is nearest to the wall.
- Lower yourself into a lunge position
  - Your right knee should be bent
  - Your left leg should be straight
  - Your left foot should be flat on the ground

- Lean toward the wall
  - You should feel a stretch in your left calf
- Hold this stretch for 30 seconds
- Repeat with the other leg

Toe Touch

- Stand with your feet shoulder width apart
- Bend forward at your waist, keeping your back straight
  - As you bend forward, allow your knees to bend slightly
- Lower your head / torso toward the floor
  - Only bend as far as you are comfortable
  - Your goal is to, over time, bend further and further toward the floor
- Hold stretch for 30 seconds
- Slowly stand back up

Shoulder Stretch

- Stand with feet shoulder width apart.
- Bring your left arm straight across your chest
- Use your right hand to pull your left arm in tight to your chest
  - Make sure your shoulders don't rise
  - Don't pull your arm at the elbow joint
- Hold stretch for 30 seconds
- Repeat with the other arm

Chest Expansion

- Stand with feet shoulder width apart
- Reach your arms behind you and clasp your hands together
- Lift your chest up, raise your arms up slightly behind you keeping them clasped
- Hold stretch for 30 seconds

Combined summary chart

	Reel Mower	Push Mower	Self-Propelled	Riding
Calories	458	288	202	86
Percent	**433%**	**235%**	**135%**	
Lowest Cost	$70	$151.15	$258.36	$1,404
Percent	**100%**	**216%**	**369%**	**20,006%**
Highest Cost	$151.15	$314.65	$560.82	$13,331.78
Percent	**216%**	**450%**	**801%**	**19,045%**

The five biggest mistakes clients make

Consistently, I see clients make the same mistakes when it comes to their health and fitness. Here are my top five:

1. Using their body weight as a measure of being overweight instead of calipers
2. Thinking setting negative goals like 'lose weight so they can fit in a pair of jeans for their class reunion' instead of forward-thinking goals like 'stronger cardiovascular health so they live a long happy life'
3. Just running. Because I already know how to run, what is there to learn?
4. Not stretching so their muscles are like tight rubber bands
5. Hiring some dipwad who took a weekend course to be their health coach or personal trainer

Get one month of free health coaching

I am so serious about helping you develop the habit of fitness mowing that I will offer you a month consisting of three 30-minute coaching sessions to help you get the habit cemented in place. As part of working together I will even send you a pair of body calipers along with instructions so you can see your progress for yourself.

All you have to do is email me a copy of the bill of sale for your riding mower along with a store receipt for purchasing your push mower.

Email your documents along with your full name, address, and phone number to sgraham@trueazimuth.biz and I'll take it from there.

Resources:

ChiRunning and ChiWalking

Danny Dreyer & Katherine Dreyer, paperback 2009
ChiRunning: A Revolutionary Approach to Effortless, Injury-Free Running

Danny Dreyer & Katherine Dreyer, paperback 2006
ChiWalking: Fitness Walking for Lifelong Health and Energy

Stretching

Jay Blahnik, paperback 2010
Full-Body Flexibility

Choosing a health coach / personal trainer

G. Scott Graham, Kindle edition 2015
Ten Things You Need to Know About Coaching Before You Get a Coach
Here's the companion website to the book:
www.howtochooseacoach.com

The Galloway Method

Jeff Galloway, paperback 2016
The Run-Walk-Run Method

Interval timers: www.gymboss.com

Scythes and scything

David Tresemer & Peter Vido, paperback (multiple editions)
The Scythe Book

Ian Miller, paperback 2016
The Scything Handbook: Learn How to Cut Grass, Mow Meadows and Harvest Grain with a Scythe

Buy a scythe: scythesupply.com

Safety considerations

While mowing your lawn is a great way to exercise, it's not without its risks.

The information presented in this book is not intended to diagnose any medical condition or to replace your healthcare professional.

You should consult your physician or other healthcare professional before starting this or any other fitness program to determine if it is right for your needs. This is particularly true if you (or your family) have a history of high blood pressure or heart disease; or if you have ever experienced chest pain when exercising or have experienced chest pain in the past month when not engaged in physical activity. Also consult them if you smoke, have high cholesterol, are obese, or have a bone or joint problem that could be made worse by a change in physical activity. Do not start this fitness program if your physician or healthcare provider advises against it. If you experience faintness, dizziness, pain or shortness of breath at any time while exercising, you should stop immediately.

Always look after yourself while mowing the lawn e.g., wear sunscreen and a hat etc.

Also make sure you drink plenty of water. The sun's heat combined with vigorous mowing dehydrates you and increases your body's heat output. This can increase the risk for heat injuries including heat exhaustion and heatstroke.

About Scott Graham

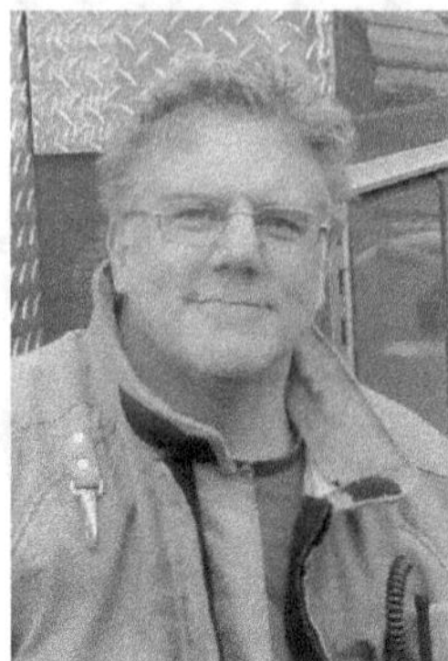

Scott is a business and career coach from Boston, MA. When he is not coaching people to be their best, he participates in Tough Mudders, hikes, works on a farm, practices Vipassana meditation, or volunteers as an EMT and firefighter.

Books by G. Scott Graham

Ten Things You Need to Know About Coaching Before You Get a Coach

Motivational Interviewing Made Easy

Work Exchange: A Handbook for Hosts

How to Become More Linkable… …and Likeable on LinkedIn

Check! Your Guide to Creating a Life Transforming Bucket List

Growing & Using Good King Henry

Make Time Your Superhero Power!

Get Off Your Ass & Mow The Grass!

Now what? After Your Vipassana Course Is Over

Determining Marijuana Use in the Age of Legalization

Androphile Pride

Treatment Planning 101

Come As You Are: Meditation & Grief

Motivational Interviewing Made Easy: Another 5 Weeks

Contact G. Scott Graham

True Azimuth, LLC
265 Franklin Street
Suite 1702
Boston, MA 02110

Phone: (617) 475-0081

Website: http://TrueAzimuth.biz. http://gscottgraham.com

Email: sgraham@TrueAzimuth.biz

Twitter: @TrueAzimuth, @grahamgscott

Goodreads: https://www.goodreads.com/grahamgscott

Facebook: http://www.facebook.com/trueazimuthcoaching,
https://www.facebook.com/author.gscottgraham

LinkedIn: http://www.linkedin.com/company/true-azimuth-llc,
https://www.linkedin.com/in/bostoncareercoach/

www.ingramcontent.com/pod-product-compliance
Lightning Source LLC
Chambersburg PA
CBHW051841250726
48659CB00005B/1960